Ichraf Jbir
Asma Belguith
Hiba Ketata

Patient well-being in intensive care

Ichraf Jbir
Asma Belguith
Hiba Ketata

Patient well-being in intensive care

The nurse's contribution to patient well-being in intensive care

ScienciaScripts

Cover image: www.ingimage.com

This book is a translation from the original published under ISBN 978-620-6-72578-7.

Publisher:
Sciencia Scripts
is a trademark of
Dodo Books Indian Ocean Ltd. and OmniScriptum S.R.L publishing group

120 High Road, East Finchley, London, N2 9ED, United Kingdom
Str. Armeneasca 28/1, office 1, Chisinau MD-2012, Republic of Moldova, Europe
Printed at: see last page
ISBN: 978-620-8-22225-3

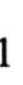

TABLE OF CONTENTS

1. INTRODUCTION

Comfort and well-being are essential for anyone hospitalised in order to regain or maintain their physical, psychological and/or mental health. This offers patients a better quality of life, particularly when they are hospitalised in an environment such as an intensive care unit [1]. This department cares for serious patients suffering from a potentially life-threatening illness or trauma. Its main objective is to ensure that patients survive with a satisfactory long-term quality of life. To meet this objective, alleviate acute visceral failure and improve the overall prognosis of these patients, a number of techniques are required (monitoring, mechanical ventilation, tracheal suctioning, artificial nutrition, etc.), as well as constant surveillance by medical and paramedical staff, which constantly generates noise (from machines, alarms, staff, other patients, etc.) and artificial light that are sources of general discomfort. These care techniques and monitoring requirements, combined with the limitations caused by the disease, loss of energy and vitality, and pain, create very difficult living conditions for patients, who are subject to numerous stress factors during their stay [1,2].

Similarly, the very mention of the word "intensive care unit" is a source of anxiety for patients, particularly because of the seriousness of the pathologies that led to their admission to these units, which are a confusing place, with many causes of psychological disturbance (lack of sleep, anxiety, thirst, etc.). In fact, almost 80% of patients admitted to intensive care admit to having had unpleasant experiences, which can lead them to react in various ways: aggression, agitation, rejection, anxiety, disorientation [3].

The challenge for the intensive care unit is to care for these serious patients in the best possible medical and technical conditions, while promoting their well-being and maintaining a high level of safety. In fact, the well-being of the intensive care patient includes both physical well-being (avoiding unnecessary suffering, making the right medical decisions) and psychological well-being (the patient's sense of well-being), prescribing the right tests, etc.) and psychological well-being (taking the person's integrity into account). As a result, well-being encompasses everything that concerns the patient and relates to good quality: quality of life for patients during their stay in intensive care, quality of care, quality of medical and paramedical care, quality of human relations [4].

In order to meet this challenge and improve the stay of patients in intensive care, it is important to preserve quality of life, reduce sources of discomfort and constantly encourage recognition of the patient as a person. The first measure to be introduced in an intensive care unit with the aim of reducing the level of discomfort perceived by patients as much as possible could be to set up a continuous assessment of potential sources of discomfort. It is possible that the awareness of each of the players, doctors and non-medical care staff, will be raised during the assessment phase, leading to a change in patient behaviour. Psychological and physical comfort must therefore be a priority in the care of these intensive care patients, and an objective of care in its own right, as it is often based on simple factors that depend on the environment and the behaviour of the carers. For this reason, and because in most intensive care units the assessment of patients' subjective symptoms is not part of daily clinical practice, we chose to address the subject of patient well-being in the intensive care unit as part of our final year project.Our main objective is to identify the discomforts experienced by patients during their stays in intensive care.Our research question is as follows: How can nursing staff contribute to reducing sources of nuisance and discomfort for patients during their stay in intensive care?In order to carry out our research, we first conducted an investigation based on literature reviews, seeking to explore concepts related to our theme, namely well-being in the context of intensive care, discomfort in intensive care and the role of carers. This stage was essential, as it enabled us to draft the problem and define the research question. Secondly, we described the research methodology that we used in developing this project, which involves a survey using a pre-established questionnaire designed to collect information on the discomfort perceived by patients during their stay in intensive care. Finally, we discussed the results obtained, followed by a conclusion including recommendations likely to improve the stay in intensive care and reduce the discomfort perceived by the patient.

2. MATERIALS AND METHOD

2.1.TYPE AND PURPOSE OF THE SURVEY :

The aim of this descriptive cross-sectional survey was to identify the discomforts experienced by patients during their stay in intensive care, with a view to analysing the role of nurses in establishing a climate of well-being.

2.2.PLACE AND DURATION OF THE ENQUIRY :

This survey took place in the central intensive care unit, A21 at Charles Nicolle Hospital and the intensive care unit at Soukra Clinic. It took place over a period of one month, from 17 January to 17 February 2020.

2.3.TARGET POPULATION :

Our work was carried out on 30 patients hospitalised in the intensive care units described above. The average length of stay was fixed at over 72 hours (3 days). The length of stay took into account the period from the date of admission to the day of discharge from the intensive care unit.

2.3.1. INCLUSION CRITERIA :

- You must be 18 or over.
- Patients admitted to one of the included intensive care units during the predetermined study period with a stay of at least 3 days.
- Patients who voluntarily agreed to answer the questions.
- Patients with preserved cognitive function on the day of the survey.

2.3.2. EXCLUSION CRITERIA :

- Under 18 years of age.
- A stay in intensive care of less than 2 days.
- Patients who refused to take part in the study.
- Patients with diminished mental capacity. A total of 30 patients were interviewed.

2.4. DATA COLLECTION TOOL :

Patient discomfort was assessed using a questionnaire inspired by the French IPREA questionnaire ("Inconforts des Patients de Reanimation"). (Appendix 1). This is a specific questionnaire for assessing patient comfort in intensive care, which has been well validated and developed using standard procedures. It has previously benefited from a feasibility study and has been validated internationally (Appendix 1). This questionnaire comprises 24 questions, 18 of which are closed and 6 multiple choice. The questions

relate to the discomforts associated with the patient and their pathology, and the environment, à organisation of work and the discomfort physical or psychological discomfort. (Appendix 2).
Interviews with patients were carried out just after discharge from the intensive care unit. To facilitate communication with the patients, we made a few modifications to the form and used the questionnaire written in Arabic (Appendix 3).

2.5.CONDUCT OF THE SURVEY :

Patients were informed in advance of the objectives and details of the study, which enabled us to obtain their oral consent. The forms used for the interview were anonymous in order to reassure the patients. Patients were informed that their answers would not influence their subsequent treatment. The interviews with the patients were carried out by us in a quiet place conducive to confidentiality. We were careful to avoid high-traffic areas and not to be disturbed during the interview. We tried to choose the right time for the interview, i.e. outside of care or meal times. We did our best to use a simple and clear vocabulary with an attitude caring and empathetic. During the interviews, we refocused the discussion on the objectives of the interview, while allowing the patient to express themselves.

2.6.DATA ANALYSIS AND ENTRY :

The data was analysed and entered using Excel software. The results were presented in the form of tables and figures, with percentages rounded up or down to make the study feasible and to facilitate statistical analysis.

2.7.ETHICAL CONSIDERATIONS :

This study was conducted with the following ethical considerations in mind Discretion in the treatment of the information given, respect for the anonymity of the participants and confidentiality. Verbal consent was obtained from each participant after the objectives of the study had been communicated. Permission was sought from the SUPSAT administration and the doctors in charge of the departments where the study was taking place to gain access to the departments and to interview patients.

2.8.LIMITATIONS OF THE STUDY :

The answers obtained are always subjective and come from a sample of patients. Consequently, the answers obtained only concern the patients surveyed. For this reason, the results of this study cannot be generalised.

3. RESULTS

3.1. EPIDEMIOLOGICAL DATA :

3.1.1. BREAKDOWN OF THE SAMPLE BY GENDER :

The sample size was 53% male and 47% female, with a sex ratio of 1.14.

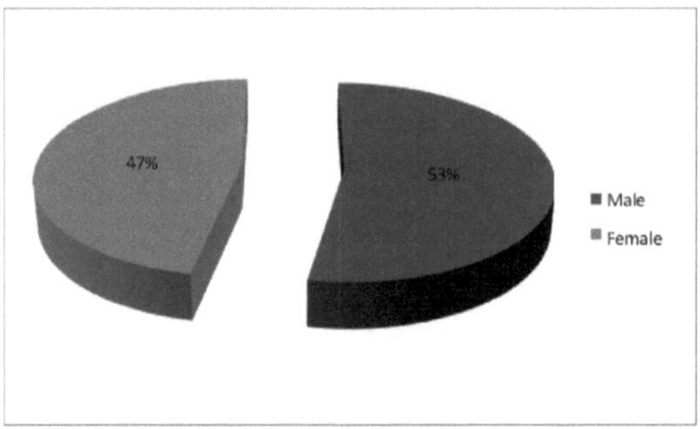

Figure 1: Breakdown of the sample by gender

3.1.2. BREAKDOWN OF THE SAMPLE BY AGE GROUP :

The average age was 58, with extremes ranging from 18 to 68. The most common age group was over 60 (47%).

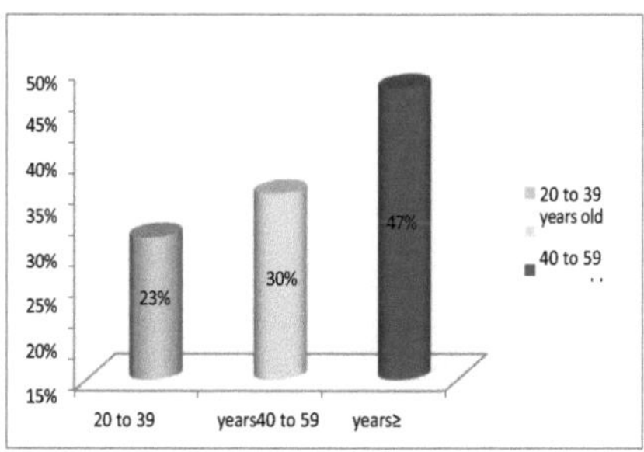

Figure 2: Breakdown of the sample by age group

3.1.3. REPARTITION OF THE SAMPLE BY THE NATURE OF HOSPITALISATION :

Two-thirds of our population were hospitalised in a surgical intensive care unit.

Table 1: Breakdown of the sample by type of hospitalisation

Type of hospitalisation	Number	Percentage
Medical	10	33%
Surgical	20	67%
Total	30	100%

3.1.4. BREAKDOWN OF THE SAMPLE BY LENGTH OF STAY IN RESUSCITATION :

The average length of stay in intensive care was 13 days, distributed as follows: One week for 40% of the population, 2 weeks for 33% and more than 3 weeks for 27%. The extremes ranged from 4 to 22 days in hospital.

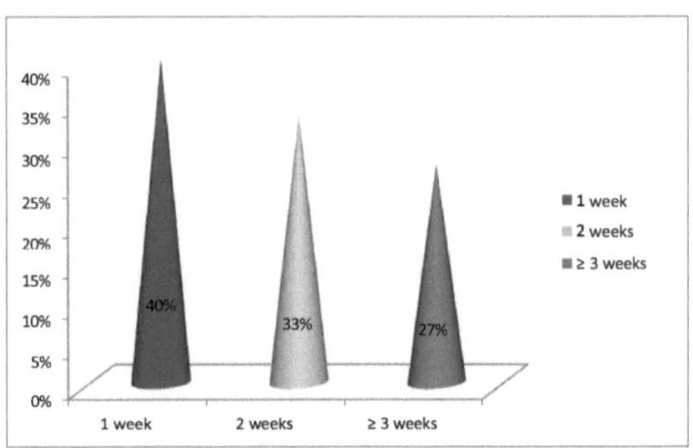

Figure 3 : Distribution of the sample by length of stay in intensive care unit

3.2. PATIENTS' FEELINGS :

3.2.1. DISCOMFORTS RELATED TO THE PATIENT AND/OR HIS/HER PATHOLOGY:

3.2.1.1.1.1. Physical discomfort :

Pain, thirst and lack of sleep were the three main causes of physical discomfort experienced by patients (93.73 and 60% respectively). Half the patients complained of hunger and 43% of them felt cold or hot (Table 2 and Figure 4).

Table 2: Physical discomforts related to the patient and/or his/her pathology

Type of discomfort	Number	Percentage
Pain	28	93%
Thirst	22	73%
Lack of sleep	18	60%
Hunger	15	50%
Heat	13	43%
Cold	13	43%

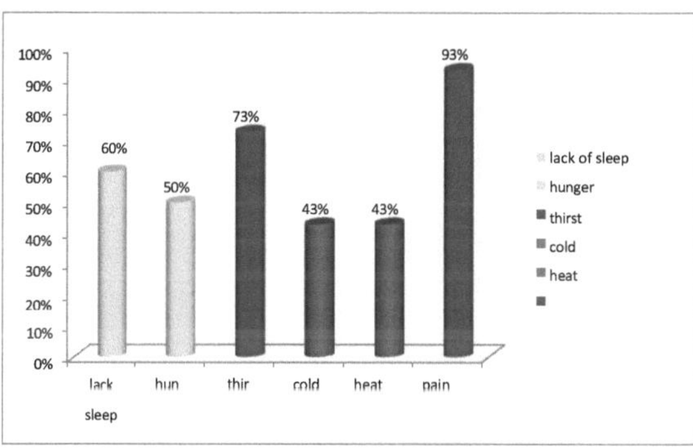

Figure 4: Distribution of sources of physical discomfort related to the patient and/or their pathology

Pain was felt more in surgical settings than in medical settings. (Table3).

Table 3: Pain experienced and hospital environment

	Medical trauma (10 patients)	Surgical recovery (20 patients)
Pain	9	19
Percentage	90%	95%

3.2.1.2. Mental discomfort

The sources of psychological discomfort were linked to a lack of respect for privacy in more than half the cases, isolation and an inability to communicate in 40% of cases, and anxiety in 37% of patients. (Table 4).

Table 4: Sources of psychological discomfort

Discomfort	Number	Percentage
Lack of respect for privacy	16	53%
Isolation	12	40%
Anguish	11	37%

The feeling of anxiety was much more intense when the hospital stay exceeded 3 weeks (Table 5).

Table 5: Anxiety and length of hospital stay

Length of hospital stay	Number	Percentage
Less than 3 weeks	4	36%
More than 3 weeks	7	64%
Total	11	100%

3.2.2. DISCOMFORTS LINKED TO THE ENVIRONMENT :

Discomfort related to the environment was linked to noise according to 83% of patients, excessive light and the poor condition of the bed according to 60% and 57% of patients respectively, and pipes according to 37% of patients. (Table 6 and Figure 5)

Table 6: Sources of discomfort linked to the environment

Discomfort	Number	Percentage
Noise	25	83%
Too much light	18	60%
Uncomfortable bed	17	57%
Surrounded by pipes	11	37%

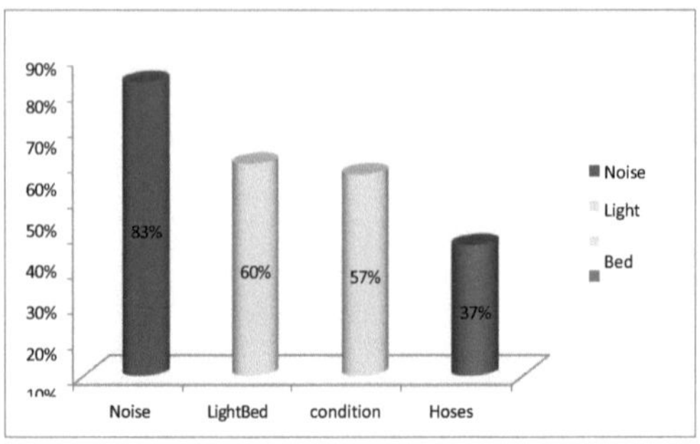

Figure 5: Distribution of sources of discomfort linked to the environment

3.2.2.1.2.1. Noise sources :

The sources of noise were the coming and going of carers according to 93% of patients, machine alarms according to 57%, conversations according to 43% and ringing telephones according to 23% of staff.

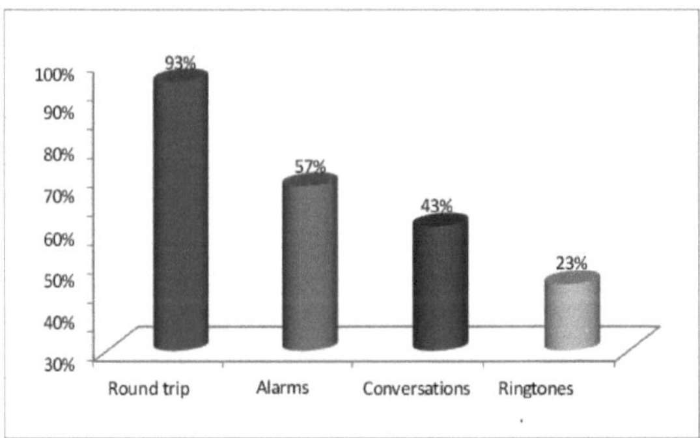

Figure 6: Noise sources

3.2.2.2. Sources of discomfort related to the state of the bed :

The discomfort caused by the state of the bed was related to **the quality of the mattress (too hard or too soft)** according to the majority of patients **(93%)** and the water mattress according to half of them.

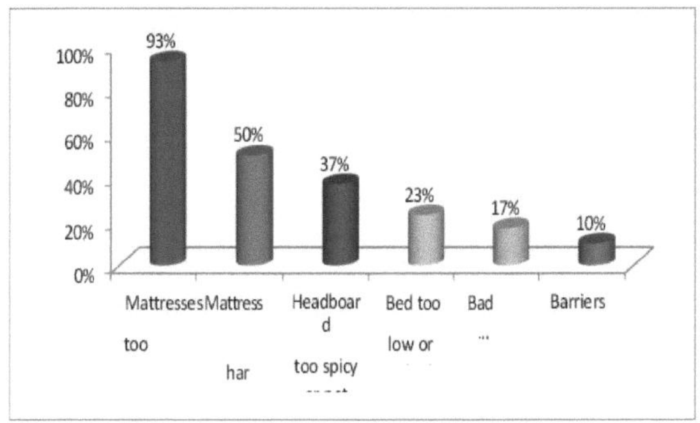

Figure 7: Sources of discomfort related to the state of the bed

3.2.2.3. Types of pipes responsible for patient discomfort :

Infusors were the main tubing responsible for patient discomfort **(67%).** Electrodes, oxygen catheters or masks and pulse oximetry were only responsible for discomfort in less than half of patients.

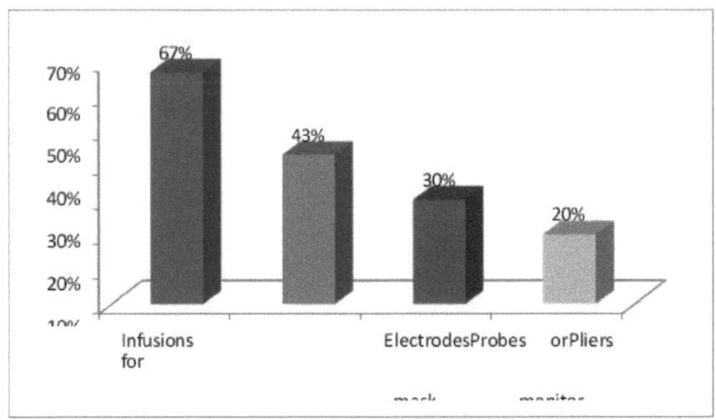

Figure 8: Types of hose responsible for patient discomfort

3.2.3. DISCOMFORTS LINKED TO WORK ORGANISATION :

3.2.3.1. Moments of lack of respect for privacy :

More than 60% of patients felt that their privacy was not respected during nappy changing and hygiene care. Nursing care and medical examinations were responsible for a lack of respect for patient privacy in less than a third of the workforce.

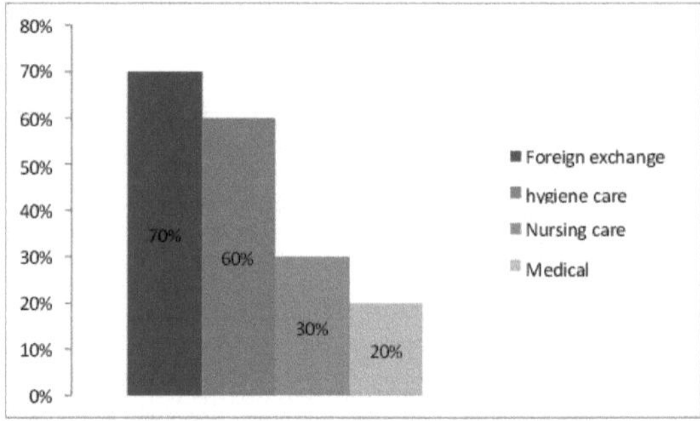

Figure 9: Moments of lack of privacy

3.2.3.2. Causes of feelings of isolation :

The poor organisation of work had led to a distressing feeling of isolation in 12 patients, i.e. 40% of the workforce. This feeling of isolation was mainly related to loneliness in the intensive care room, according to 9 patients (Figure 10).

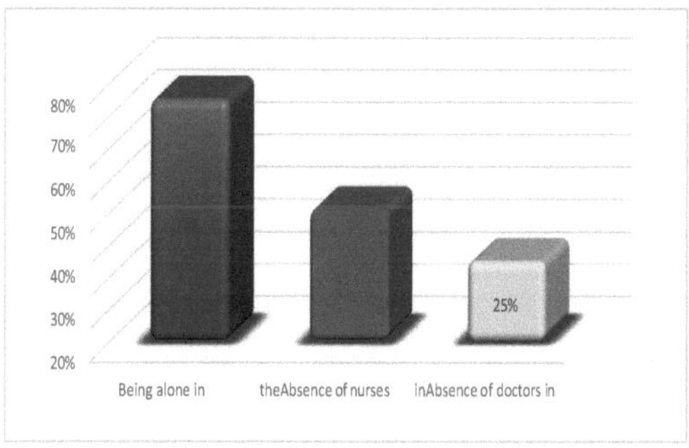

Figure 10: Causes of feelings of isolation

3.2.3.3. Lack of information

The lack of information concerned the steps to be taken and the course of the disease, according to almost half the patients.

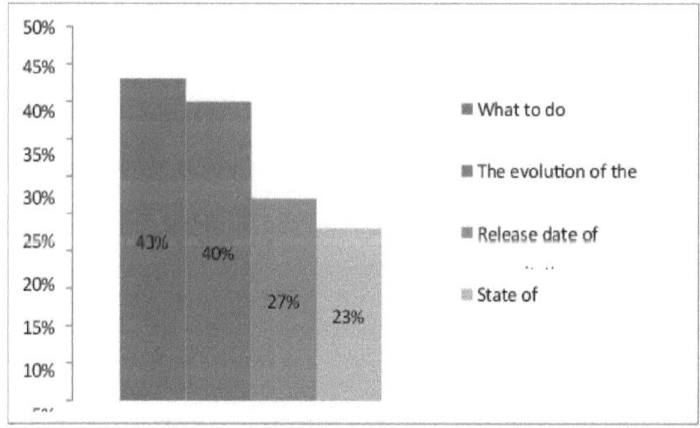

Figure 11: Lack of information

3.2.3.4. Limiting visits from family and friends:

Of the 30 patients surveyed, 14 (47%) were bothered by the reduction in visits from family members. These patients reported that this limitation on visiting hours aggravated their feelings of isolation and lack of communication.

4. DISCUSSION

The aim of this study was to identify the discomfort experienced by patients during their stay in intensive care. To this end, we conducted a survey of a sample of patients immediately after their discharge from the intensive care unit.

4.1. EPIDEMIOLOGICAL STUDY :

More than half of our sample was represented by male patients (53%) with an average age of 58 years. This result is consistent with a retrospective study conducted in the polyvalent intensive care unit of the Fattouma Bourguiba Hospital in Monastir, Tunisia, between 1 September 2012 and 31 August 2013. The aim of this retrospective study was to assess pain in intensive care patients. It included 279 patients, 63% of whom were male with an average age of 56 years. This allows us to conclude that our sample has epidemiological characteristics similar to those of the Monastir study and could be representative of all intensive care patients in Tunisia [5].

4.2. PATIENTS' FEELINGS :

In our study, all the patients surveyed experienced physical or psychological discomfort linked either to their pathology, or to the environment or organisation of work in the intensive care unit. This is consistent with a recent French study which showed that the sources of discomfort remain identical. Pain, sleep deprivation, thirst, immobilisation by infusions and cables, noise and anxiety obtained the highest scores for the intensity of discomfort generated [6].

4.3.DISCOMFORTS RELATED TO THE PATIENT AND/OR HIS/HER PATHOLOGY :

With regard to discomforts linked to the patient and their pathology, our study showed that they were linked to pain (93%), thirst (73%) and sleep deprivation. (60%). These results suggest that pain in intensive care is one of the main sources of discomfort for patients.

4.3.1. PAIN AND ITS MANAGEMENT :

In the literature, the pathologies that lead patients to the ICU (polytrauma, surgery, pancreatitis, etc.) and the ICU itself (catheters, mechanical ventilation, etc.) are sources of pain [7]. Half of patients hospitalised in intensive care develop moderate to severe pain, whether the reason for admission is postoperative, traumatic or a medical pathology. In our series, the pain was more severe in the surgical setting than in the medical setting. This could be related to the pain of surgical wounds, but our questionnaire did not take into account the sources of pain. In this respect, several studies have found that "many patients report high pain scores for all care procedures: lateral positioning, central line insertions, drain removals, wound dressings, tracheal aspirations, femoral catheter removals, intubation tubes" [8,6]. According to a French national survey conducted between 5 January 2004 and 31 January 2005, which included 1,381 patients recruited from 44 intensive care centres, pain in intensive care is frequent and intense. Five days after discharge from intensive care, 63% of patients described their pain as moderate to severe. Nearly half of the patients said that they had experienced pain during their stay in intensive care, and 15% of them described their pain as severe. In our work, the questionnaire did not qualify the intensity of the pain [9].

- **Pain management :**

Nurses should alleviate the pain associated with care by respecting patients' safety, communicating with them and being gentle. Failing that, they may resort to the use of pharmaceutical products on medical prescription.In all cases, nursing staff must focus their care not only on the illness and the techniques used to support it, but also on the patient, who must be considered as human beings. In this respect, several authors have shown that "Talking with them" is the basic principle of caring for a patient who is recognised as a human being [9, 10].

4.3.2. Sleep deprivation and its management :

This study showed that patients complained of sleep deprivation in 60% of cases. This lack of sleep was related to the patient and his or her pathology (algic, anxious patients). According to a French national survey, pain, lack of sleep, anxiety, nightmares and hallucinations were the most unpleasant memories, evoked by almost 70% of patients [9], Furthermore, in the intensive care setting, the technical nature of the care provided and the safety and monitoring requirements also compromise sleep quality. In this context, a French study using 24-hour polysomnographic recording showed that intensive care patients slept for an average of 5 hours, and that the duration of non-waking sleep episodes was just 3 minutes [2]. The same study highlighted the poor quality of sleep caused by noise pollution, the number of treatments and excessive light intensity.

➢ **Managing sleep deprivation :**

The literature reports that the role of good quality sleep on health is recognised [11]. Nursing staff should therefore take action to combat patients' physical and mental suffering, which are major sources of sleep deprivation, by prescribing analgesics and anxiolytics. It is also essential to limit interruptions to sleep at night by reducing light and the volume of alarms, and by grouping care activities together.

4.3.3. THIRST :

In our series, thirst was a major source of discomfort in 73% of cases. A recent French study of more than 1,500 post-operative cardiac surgery patients, based on the administration of a post-anaesthesia complaints and satisfaction questionnaire developed by the German Society for Intensive Care Anaesthesia, showed that 85% of patients complained of thirst and dry mouth, and 60% of patients complained of pain at the surgical site [12]. According to the same study, other sources of discomfort need to be taken into account on a daily basis, such as hunger, cold, feelings of isolation or even dependence and vulnerability [12].

4.4. ENVIRONMENTAL DISCOMFORTS :

4.4.1. NOISE AND ITS MANAGEMENT :

The World Health Organisation (WHO) recommends an ambient noise level of less than 35 decibels (dB) for adequate rest at night [11]. In the present study, 83% of the respondents were bothered by noise, the sources of which were the coming and going of carers (93%), machine alarms (57%), conversations between carers (43%) and ringing telephones (23%).These results show that, on the one hand, noise is recognised as a source of discomfort during a stay in an intensive care unit and, on the other hand, certain sources of noise can be avoided by good management of alarms and the adoption of appropriate behaviour by carers. In this respect, the literature reports that calm in intensive care units is essential for the well-being of patients, who are often surrounded by therapeutic and diagnostic procedures such as intubation, gastric or bladder catheters, pleural drainage and central and peripheral venous catheters connected to infusions [4]. Nurses should therefore mobilise patients and remove all catheters, cables and probes as soon as possible when they are no longer required. This helps patients to see the improvement in their state of health.

4.4.2. EXCESS LIGHT AND ITS MANAGEMENT:

In our study, 60% of the patients surveyed were bothered by excessive light, both day and night. In this respect, several studies have shown that limiting light sources, particularly at night, facilitates the reestablishment of a sleep-wake cycle and should be a priority for the comfort and well-being of intensive care patients [13, 14]. To reduce excess light, the nursing staff must keep the bedroom doors closed if the patient so wishes, make a light source available to the patient and keep the doors open. pocket per room for night-time surveillance to be used by carers and doctors, close the blinds or curtains according to the patient's wishes and dim the lights on the ward and in each room at night.

4.4.3. Pipe gene :

Several studies have used the subjective approach to assess discomfort perceived by patients. In theory, this approach is simple to implement, since it is based on questionnaires submitted to patients. In the first study, the presence of tubes through the mouth or nose were the discomforts most often cited by patients [15]. In the second study, carried out on a very small population of patients in a single intensive care unit to classify the 40 sources of 'stress', six discomforts were associated with a high score. These six discomforts were, in addition to "having pain" and "not being able to sleep", "having tubes in the nose or mouth", "being attached by cables and infusion lines", "not having self-control" and "not receiving explanations about treatments received" [16]. In our study, which is also based on a questionnaire for intensive care patients, 37% had experienced discomfort related to being surrounded by tubes, with infusion lines being considered a major source of discomfort in 67% of cases. The nursing staff should then remove all the tubes surrounding the patient as soon as possible (infusers, probes, catheters, electrodes), enabling them to see the early improvement in their state of health, which is a major source of psychological comfort.

4.4.4. DISCOMFORT DUE TO THE STATE OF THE BED:

In the present study, 57% of respondents were bothered by the uncomfortable state of the bed, the sources of which were the quality of the mattress in 93% of cases and the water mattress according to half of the sample. This type of discomfort has not been described in the literature.

4.5. DISCOMFORTS ASSOCIATED WITH WORK ORGANISATION :

Our patients surveyed mentioned discomforts linked to the poor organisation of the work, such as the reduction in visiting times, the lack of information and the feeling of isolation due to the solitude in the intensive care room and the absence of a nurse nearby. A French study carried out in 2008 reported that patient discomfort in the intensive care unit is increased by the lack of explanations given to the patient, as well as the poor organisation of care and the unavailability of staff. The same study also reported that vulnerable patients who are dependent and unable to communicate feel isolated [17]. These factors make it more difficult to detect discomfort and are described as stressful. Similarly, our study concluded that the lack of information, particularly about what to do and how their disease was progressing, further increased the feeling of discomfort.Another French study, based on a questionnaire submitted to intensive care patients, reported that, in addition to sleep deprivation, the inability to communicate and the limitation of visits were the discomforts most complained about by the patients studied [18].

➢ What can be done to improve the organisation of work in intensive care?

Nurses should make it easier for patients to visit their families and extend their visiting hours, as family visits can help to detect and reduce anxiety disorders in patients. In this respect, the literature agrees that the more the family feels "good", the more they will be able to help the patient feel "better". " [2, 11]. As a result, the well-being of relatives becomes an essential part of the patient's well-being. Staff must comfort and reassure patients' families. Similarly, nurses should concentrate on providing care and avoid personal conversations between carers and patients. As for the patient, if his condition allows it, he must be informed of the actions to be taken and the progress of his condition. In fact, the quality of communication with the patient is a criterion for judging his or her well-being, because the human approach is essential and involves attitudes, gestures and words of compassion and reassurance. Consequently, the care team must pay close attention to communication with the patient, whatever their condition, and must maintain contact with them at all times by explaining and alerting them to the care being provided, including in the case of patients who are sedated or who have been sedated. unconscious. This contact can be ensured either through verbal or non-verbal communication. In addition to verbal communication, non-verbal communication plays an even more important role when there are significant physical constraints (intubation, artificial ventilation, etc.), using methods of communication that give priority to touch, look and voice. In this respect, another study has shown that "it is through non-verbal communication, even during major visceral failures, that supportive actions such as encouragement, attention and reassurance, all of which are desired by patients, will be most effective" [19].

4.6. PSYCHOLOGICAL DISCOMFORT :

Physical care, including nursing and physiotherapy, allows patients to reinvest in their bodies. On the other hand, handling that is too mechanical and cold, and that does not respect the patient's intimacy, can be felt as a physical as well as a psychological aggression [2]. In our series, 53% of patients reported a lack of respect for privacy, particularly during diaper changes and hygiene care, according to more than 60% of patients. During this care, nurses must respect this intimacy so as not to aggravate the patient's condition by causing psychological trauma combined with physical suffering. In addition to the lack of respect for privacy, the pain associated with care, as well as noise and excessive light, can cause psychological disorders in intensive care patients, particularly anxiety and anguish. This was the case for 37% of our patients. This disorder was seen as a source of discomfort for some patients. The treatment of anxiety and anguish relies on verbal contact and reassurance. If this proves insufficient, an anxiolytic should be prescribed. In the literature, prolonged hospital stays have been identified as a source of stress in intensive care patients [20-21]. Similarly, in our study, 64% of anxious patients had a prolonged stay in intensive care (> 3 weeks). According to the data in the literature, it is difficult to establish a precise definition of the length of stay at which an ICU stay should be considered prolonged. In particular, there is a degree of heterogeneity depending on the type of intensive care unit considered. For example, in a cardiac surgical intensive care unit, a stay may be considered prolonged if it lasts more than three to seven days [20]. However, for medical, surgical and general intensive care units, a duration of 14 days appears to be relatively consensual and is frequently adopted [21]. As a result, the length of stay in intensive care is an important tool for assessing the quality of care and activity in an intensive care unit. The challenge for the practitioner is to ensure optimal patient care on a daily basis with the shortest possible length of stay.

5. RECOMMENDATIONS

At end of analysis of results of our study, we propose the following recommendations:

- Providing intensive care units with sufficient nursing staff so that nurses can find the time to look after patients' well-being and comfort.

- The introduction of protocols for assessing the sources of discomfort associated with hospitalisation in an intensive care unit, using a subjective approach based on questionnaires submitted by nursing staff.

- Development of an approach to improving patient well-being, which must be supported by line managers (the department's head doctor and the nurse in charge) in order to promote it and motivate the entire care team to apply it.

- The creation within each intensive care unit of a policy to reduce discomfort in the intensive care unit and a culture shared by all members of the health care team, with the indissociable objectives of patient well-being and safety.

- Raising the awareness of each carer to change their behaviour towards intensive care patients, such as controlling conversations and combating noise and excessive light.

- Raising nurses' awareness of the importance of the psychological side of patients, through good communication with patients and respect for their privacy.

6. CONCLUSION

This study identified the discomforts experienced by patients during their stay in intensive care following a survey of 30 patients after their discharge from intensive care, using a questionnaire inspired by the French IPREA questionnaire ("Inconforts des Patients de REAnimation"). Although the patients' responses are subjective, the results obtained largely reflect the reality on the ground. The main discomforts mentioned by patients following their stay in intensive care were pain (93%), noise (83%), thirst (73%), too much light (60%), lack of sleep (60%), the state of the bed (57%) and lack of privacy (53%). Reducing discomfort in intensive care therefore involves measuring the various sources of discomfort, which means identifying them beforehand and defining and validating the most appropriate measurement tools. Identifying the sources of discomfort can help carers to determine effective measures to reduce discomfort and improve patients' conditions in intensive care. The aim is to improve the environment, to take into account the symptoms most frequently reported by patients, and to organise and direct care to improve comfort. Similarly, measuring the quality of life of intensive care patients must become a daily practice in order to help establish a climate of well-being for patients. This can lead to a change in the practices of carers and an improvement in the hospitalisation conditions specific to each intensive care unit. As a result, taking into account the patient's well-being and comfort depends on the existence of a culture shared by all members of the team and real collaboration between doctors, nurses and care assistants. As far as the care team is concerned, the implementation of a discomfort reduction programme combined with a systematic assessment of the patient's genes can have a direct influence on their behaviour. Indeed, carers could make more effort than usual, which would enable them to take better account of the discomfort felt by the patient and the potential sources of discomfort. Carers should always remember that resuscitation patients need compassion, encouragement, reassurance and ongoing moral support.Doing this work has given us great comfort, because we've highlighted the discomforts felt by patients. This can be useful to us in our professional lives, where we will work to prevent discomfort in order to promote patient comfort as far as possible. Finally, this study has attempted to address the well-being of patients, but the well-being of ICU staff remains to be studied. This deserves another study.

7. BIBLIOGRAPHICAL REFERENCES

1. Béras A. Comfort of the patient in file:///C:/Documents%20and%20Settings/lg133779/Mes%20documents/Downloads/confo rt-du- patient-en-rea-chartres-1.pdf. Accessed on 25/01/2020.

2. Vinatier I. Patient well-being in intensive care: how can it be improved? Intensive care .2010 ;20(2) :662-8.

3. Schelling G,Stoll CH, Haller M, Briegel J, Manert W, Hummel Th, et al. Health-related quality of life and post-traumatic stress disorder in survivors of the acute respiratory distress syndrome.Crit Care Med 1998 ;26 :651-9.

4. Ferré F., Fourcade O. Well-being in intensive care: a common interest. Update conference .2013. [Online] : fourcade.o@chu-toulouse.fr. Accessed on 25/01/2020.

5. Dachraoui F, May I,Ouanes Z, Hammouda R, Bouzgarrou S, Bilel I, Miendel I, Touil S, Ben Abdallah L, Ouanes-Besbes, Abroug F. Typologie et devenir des patients admis en réanimation . Réanimation polyvalente. CHU F-Bourguiba,Monastir , Tunisie .2013.

6. Kalfon P, Mimoz O, Auquier P. Devlopment and validation of a questionnaire for quantitative assessment of percieved discomforts in critically ill patients. Intensive care Med.2010 ;10 :1751-8.

7. Chanques G, Sebbane M, Barbotte E, Viel E, Elediam JJ, Jaber S. A prospective study of pain at rest: incidence and characteristics of an unrecognized symptom in surgical and trauma versus medical intensive care unit patients. Anesthesiology 2007 ;107 :858-60.

8. Barr J, Fraser GL. Clinical practice guidelines for the management

of pain, agitation, and delirium in adult patients in the intensive care unit.Crit Care Med.2013 ;41 :263-306.

9. Payen JF, Rolland C, Genty C, Bosson JL. Pain in intensive care. Department of Anaesthesia and Intensive Care. Centre d'Investigation Clinique. France .2005.

10. Grosclaude M. Réanimation et coma. Soin psychique et vécu du patient .2e èd. ElsevierMasson, Paris .2009.

11. Martin C. Mieux vivre la réanimation. Conférence de consenus. Annales françaises d'anesthésie et de réanimation N°29(4).2010 :321-330.

12. Huppe M. The Anaesthesiological Questionnaire for patients in cardiac anaesthesia results of a multicenter survery bu the scientific working group for cardiac anaesthesia of the German Society for Anaesthesiology and Intensive care medicine. Anaesthesist .2005 ;54 :655-66.

13. Venhard JC, Orillard M, Perrotin D,Souhet G. Study of noise in an intensive care unit. Rean Urg .2007 ;5 :613-9.

14. Elliot R, Mckinley S, Cistulli P, Fien M. Characterisation of sleep in intensive care using 24 hour polysomnography: an observational study. Crit Care .2013 ;17 : R46.

15. Nelson JE. Self-reported symptom experience of critically ill cancer patients receiving intensive care. Crit Care Med.2001 ;29 :277-82.

16. Ballard KS. Identification of environmental stressors for patients in surgical intensive care unit. Issues Ment Health Nurs.1981 ;3 :89-108.

17. Matiti MR, Trorey GM.Patients' expectations of the maintenance of their dignity J Clin Nurs

October 2008 ;17(20) :2709-17.

18. Kamdar BB, King LM. The effect of a quality improvement intervention on percieved sleep quality and cognition in a medical ICU.Crit Care Med .2013 ;41 :800-9.

19. Pochard F. Reconnaitre et traiter la souffrance psychique en réanimation. Réanimation .2010 ;19 :236-42.

20. Hassan A, Anderson C, Kypson A. Clinical outcomes in patients with prolonged intensive care unit length of stay after cardiac surgical procedures. Ann Thorac Surg.2012 ;93 :565-9.

21. Zampieri FG, Ladeira JP, Park M. Admission factors associated with prolonged (>14 days) intensive care unit stay. J Crit Care. 2014;29 :60-5.

8. APPENDICES

APPENDIX 1: IPREA QUESTIONNAIRE

(Discomforts of Intensive Care Patients)

1. Have you suffered from noise (alarms, radios, ringing phones, conversations) day and night?
2. Have you suffered from light pollution (too much light in the bedroom or corridor, especially at night)?
3. Did you suffer in bed (mattress too hard or too soft, water mattress, headboard too high or not high enough, bed too low or too high, barriers, bad pillows, etc.)?
4. Have you suffered from a lack of sleep compared to usual?
5. Have you suffered from thirst?
6. Have you suffered from hunger?
7. Have you suffered from the cold?
8. Have you suffered from the heat?
9. Did you have any pain, even if it was present prior to hospitalisation, including pain associated with injections or during diaper changes or morning bathing?
10.did you suffer from being surrounded by tubes (for infusions, connections of electrodes fixed to the chest, oxygen in the nose or on the mask, the tongs for
monitor oxygenation, etc.)?
11. Were you bothered by the fact that your privacy was not sufficiently respected (e.g. during morning toileting, nappy changing,

examinations by doctors, or medical visits)?

12. Did you suffer from anxiety (a sometimes panicky fear, for example, that an important piece of equipment was malfunctioning, sometimes provoked by the sounding of alarms) or did you feel very anxious during your stay in hospital?

13. Have you suffered from isolation (being alone in your room, sometimes without seeing nurses or doctors nearby, and without hearing any noise)?

14. Have you been inconvenienced by the restriction on visits from family members or friends in accordance with the visiting hours in force on the ward?

15. Were you embarrassed not to have a telephone in the room?

16. Were you embarrassed by not being sufficiently informed about your condition or what was going to be done to you, how your illness was progressing, when you would be discharged from intensive care and what would happen afterwards, either by the nurses or the doctors?

A feasibility study was first carried out on this questionnaire, which was then validated and published.

APPENDIX 2 QUESTIONNAIRE ON PATIENT WELL-BEING IN INTENSIVE CARE

As part of our work, we carried out a survey **on "patient well-being in intensive care".** This questionnaire was aimed at patients who had spent more than 3 days in intensive care. It enabled us to collect data relating to our study.

A- Characteristics of respondents :

1. Genre: Male □Féminin □
2. Age years
3. Type of hospitalisation: medical □chirurgicale □
4. Length of stay in intensive care :

B- Patients' feelings :

1. Do you suffer from noise both day and night? Yes □non □
2. What do you think was the source of the noise?

A. Alarms □

B. Return journey for carers □

C. Ringtones □

D. Conversations □

3. Did you suffer from light pollution (too much light in the bedroom or corridor, especially at night)? yes □non □
4. Did you suffer from the state of the bed? yes □non □
5. What was the cause of your suffering from the state of the bed?

A. Mattress too hard or too soft □

B. Waterbed □

C. Headboard raised too high or too low □

D.Bed too low or too high □

E. Barriers □

F. Bad pillows □

6. Have you suffered from a lack of sleep compared to usual? yes □no

7. Have you suffered from thirst? yes □non □

8. Have you suffered from hunger? yes □non □

9. Did you suffer from cold? yes □non □

10.Did you suffer from heat? yes □non □

11.Did you suffer from pain? yes □non□

Have you suffered from being surrounded by pipes? yes □non □

12. What types of pipe did you find inconvenient?

A.Infusions □

B.Electrodes □

C.Oxygen probes or masks □

D.The clamp for monitoring oxygenation □

13. Were you bothered by the fact that your privacy was not sufficiently respected? yes □non □

14. At what point did you feel that your privacy was not respected?

A.During hygiene care (washing) □

B.Foreign exchange □

C.Care provided by nurses □

D.Examination by doctors □

15. Did you suffer f r o m anguish or anxiety during your hospitalisation? yes □non□

16. Have you suffered from isolation? yes □non □

17. What were the sources of your isolation?

A. Being alone in your room □

B. No nurses nearby □

C. No doctors nearby □

18. Were you inconvenienced by the restriction on visits from family members or friends according to the visiting hours in force on the ward? Yes □non □ 20.Were you bothered by the fact that you were not given enough information by nurses or other staff?doctors :

A. Your state of health	yes □	no □
B. What we were going to do to you	yes □	no □
C. The course of your illness	yes □	no □
D. Your date of discharge from intensive care	yes □	no □

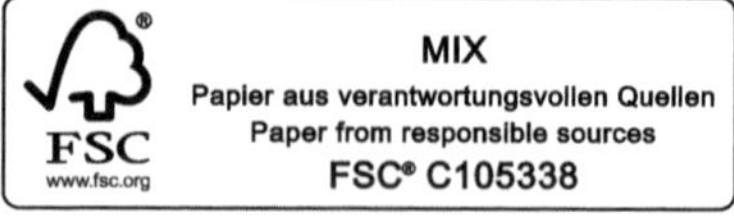

Printed by Books on Demand GmbH, Norderstedt / Germany